The Hidden Truths
About Preventing Cancer

The Hidden Truths About Preventing Cancer

A SIMPLE HANDBOOK

by

Lexie Ross

Copyright © 2016 Lexie Ross, EarthSong Publishing
All rights reserved.

ISBN-13: 9780692709191
ISBN-10: 0692709193

Table of Contents

Part One	**Cancer Causing Toxins**	1
Chapter 1	The Causes of Cancer	2
Chapter 2	The State of our Medical Profession	7
Chapter 3	Dr. Max Gerson	11
Chapter 4	Avoiding Breast Cancer	14
Chapter 5	Pesticides	16
Chapter 6	The Whole Truth About Tobacco	18
Chapter 7	Alcohol Related Cancers	21
Chapter 8	Sugar and the Loss of Will	24
Chapter 9	Aspartame	28
Chapter 10	Fluoridation	32
Chapter 11	Avoiding Microwaved Foods - Even for Coffee & Tea	35
Chapter 12	Toxic Ingredients	38
Chapter 13	MSG	41
Chapter 14	Food Coloring	46
Chapter 15	Wheat & Gluten	49
Chapter 16	Dairy Products	51
Chapter 17	Cosmetic Toxins	55

Chapter 18	Vaccines	58
Chapter 19	Electronic Pollution	61
Part Two	**Building the Immune System**	65
Chapter 20	The Importance of Drinking Pure Water	66
Chapter 21	Proper Breathing	70
Chapter 22	Fresh, Locally Grown Foods Contain Vital Enzymes	73
Chapter 23	The Challenge of Proper Food Combining	78
Chapter 24	Support For the Immune System	83
Chapter 25	The Healing Power of Vitamin C	85
Chapter 26	Colloidal Silver and Its Antibiotic Properties	87
Chapter 27	Colon Cleansing	91
Chapter 28	Medicinal Spices Used in Cooking	93
	Epilogue	99

In 1776, Dr. Benjamin Rush,
a signer of the Declaration of Independence said:

"Unless we put medical freedom into the Constitution the time will come when medicine will organize itself into an undercover dictatorship. To restrict the art of healing to doctors and deny equal privileges to others will constitute the Bastille of medical science. All such laws are un-American and despotic."

In 1953, after the healing of his son through alternative methods, Congressman Charles Tobey sponsored an investigation into what he felt was a conspiracy against the alternative medical profession. But, he conveniently died and the investigation was halted. He was among the many, many doctors and people in authority whose strange deaths occurred after prescribing alternative methods or introducing the truth about various cancer alternatives that threaten the country's cancer industry profits.

In 1964, the FDA, Food and Drug Administration spent millions to suppress alternative treatments that had cured thousands of cancer patients. In collusion, the AMA, American Medical Association and the American Cancer Society developed their own hit lists to prevent holistic doctors from actually healing cancer without using the current barbaric methods of radiation and chemotherapy. Many of these alternative doctors were either jailed, killed, their practices burned down and destroyed or they were forced to move to Mexico. The allopathic industry as a whole completely denies the opportunities for natural healing. But, in spite of their pharmaceutical/medical cartel, there is a growing number of allopathic doctors who are refusing to follow ranks. They are using alternatives to completely heal cancer and other so-called incurable diseases without causing pain and suffering. Amidst this evil dominance over the medical industry, pharmaceutical giants prefer profit over prevention or saving lives. They continue to use poisonous additives in our foods and eliminate any doctors who are healing diseases naturally, especially cancer and Lymes Disease. With the recent knowledge that over 30 holistic doctors have been murdered who were completely healing cancer, it is to them I dedicate this book.

Part One

Cancer Causing Toxins

CHAPTER 1

THE CAUSES OF CANCER

FIFTY YEARS AGO, THE INCIDENCE of cancer was so rare people were shocked when it occurred. Today, having cancer has become an accepted part of our lives. Every other person in the U.S. will have some kind of cancer, which is a horrifying reality as to the quality of life in America.

Most of us don't stop to ask what is causing so much cancer. We need to learn more about the toxic additives in our foods, medicines, water and air that are making us ill. We're so used to hearing about cancer or thinking we should be "taking something" for headaches, stomach aches, back pain, indigestion, etc. we don't identify them as warning signals. We merely assume that our diseased plight is natural. Too many of us think, "Oh Well, I'll eventually have a heart attack, develop diabetes or arthritis, have a stroke, etc, it's part of life." In reality, unless we have abused our bodies in some way, we shouldn't be in pain or discomfort at all, there is always a dietary or environmental reason.

Some of us are aware there are toxic chemicals and pesticides in our food and environment, but we don't stop to identify them or even to ask about the amounts we're imbibing. Nor do we ever consider how long it takes for these small amounts of toxins to finally reach intolerable levels that take a toll on our health. We need to identify what we are being exposed to that's causing so much cancer and other new so called "incurable" diseases like Attention Deficit Disorder, Autism, MS, Chronic Fatigue, Epstein Barr and Fibromyalgia. Or even Morgellons and Mersa, the frightening bacterial diseases people are contracting in hospitals. There is no explanation for how they surface, other than the over use of antibiotics.

No one tells us what chemicals are used in the making of the chemotherapy being injected in our bodies that cause such disastrous side affects, or the chemicals used in the manufacturing of vaccines. These chemical additives and medications are obviously weakening our organs, especially our brains, liver and kidneys. All we have to do is hear the insane litany of side affects on TV drug commercials to know that we are at risk. There simply is no long term testing, and doctors tend to deny the possibility of future complications. They don't take into consideration that every body is different. And, the FDA waits until various drugs cause deaths in numbers, or are the cause of other diseases before they are pulled off the market. We are simply not asking enough questions of the FDA and the law makers who are supposed to be safe-guarding our food system and our environment. We need to become aware of how and where our system is failing us and what can we do about it. And finally, we need to learn what ongoing choices we can make to improve our own chances of maintaining good health.

As I began to reflect on my own family history, I realized, that despite their disdain toward me for trying to guide them into a more holistic approach to life, I was the only one who hadn't developed cancer, or had my gall bladder removed - and that included my daughter. As a holistic cancer researcher, I'd been practicing the health tips that I've learned along the way and they were obviously working.

Preventing cancer is about education. I've avoided those things I knew would be harmful to my body beginning with: severely limiting my intake of processed foods, avoiding fast food restaurants, avoiding the use of microwave ovens, not drinking tap water, choosing healthy cooking oils and choosing soaps and cosmetics that do not contain harmful chemicals. For the last 40 years, my philosophy has been to eat fresh, live and if possible, organic food. If you stick with these suggestions, are not addicted to alcohol, cigarettes or sugar, and you avoid other food and cosmetic toxins, unless you are exposed to some environmental poison through your job or are enduring some kind of physically or emotionally toxic environment, you should be able to maintain your health.

My sagely mother developed cancer, but she healed it twice with a combination of juices she concocted she said were given to her by God. I've always deeply regretted having not written down her formula. That was before I became a holistic journalist.

When she healed herself twice with her juice combination, her doctor was amazed, but never bothered to ask her for the formula either. Both of my sisters died of cancer and despite my counseling, my daughter allowed doctors to convince her that she needed a double mastectomy for a small tumor in her left breast that could have easily been healed. Not only did her doctor tell her if she removed her breasts, she would be completely healed of her cancer, he told her they wouldn't remove her lymph nodes, which they did.

Shortly afterward, due to complications, she had to have two more brutally painful surgeries and then a few years later, she had three more surgeries, all related to the side effects that developed after her initial surgery. As a teenager, she had been in a car accident with every bone in her body being broken, but she said nothing was as horrible as the pain she endured with her radical mastectomy and the two other operations that ensued. Thankfully, she refused to take the chemo, radiation and tamoxifen they suggested.

I'm appalled when I talk to women who were persuaded by their doctors to have their breasts cut off or when they haven't yet developed the disease and are frightened into costly, painful surgery as a preventive. I was particularly furious when one of my young friends who didn't even have cancer was coerced to have both breasts cut off while she was in her thirties because her aunt had gotten cancer. The doctors grafted skin from her back to build her new breasts. She said the pain was like military torture.

Back in the 70's, when I saw the bald, dying, death-gray children in their wheel chairs outside of Sloan Kettering hospital in New York, it brought tears to my eyes. I became furious to think that anyone would allow children or adults to suffer such barbaric procedures. I knew God had to have more gentle, pain-free ways to heal cancer and I became determined to find them. I say them, because there are many cures, but they are carefully kept out of the market place by the pharmaceutical industry that finances most of the medical schools in America.

In the following pages, I list the major toxins to avoid, and then provide some of the positive things you can do to help you enhance your overall health.

CHAPTER 2

The State of our Medical Profession

~~~~~~

First of all, cancer is not a death sentence, it's a signal that the body is out-of-balance. When people tell me they have been diagnosed with cancer and look scared to death, I explain to them that in many cases, it can be cured with just a lifestyle change. But they have been so frightened and brainwashed by their doctors, they tend not to believe me. There is now a significant body of evidence proving that people who avoid chemo, radiation and radical mastectomy live longer than those who are convinced by their doctors to undergo these debilitating treatments. If you are given a cancer diagnosis, by all means get a second or even a third opinion.

Cancer is a two hundred billion dollar industry and the prescription drug companies that train doctors, are not interested in finding a cure. In fact, Big Pharma conducts workshops in medical schools convincing doctors that alternative medicine is quackery. Their first priority is selling drugs, increasing profits and pleasing stock holders.

The cancer industry as a whole acts on the "Kill Principle" as opposed to finding gentle ways to stimulate the body's own immune system. In light of the suffering caused by chemo and radiation and how much damage it does to the whole body, it's shocking to hear that today's doctors are not trained to help you become well, or to introduce any kind of preventive methods that would keep cancer from happening, it simply isn't as profitable.

At a medical conference in New York, one of my doctor friends overheard the director of one of the leading cancer hospitals say, "If God placed the cure for cancer in my hand today, I'd toss it in the waste paper basket."

Ralph Moss, former Marketing Director of Sloan Kettering hospital in New York gives an honest assessment of allopathic medicine in his book, *The Cancer Industry*. He explains that the allopathic health industry removed any kind of prevention out of the medical schools in the 1980's. Instead, they encourage the more costly use of radiation and chemotherapy, in addition to scheduling patients for unnecessary MRI's and Cat Scans. He explains that hospitals really don't need more than one MRI or CAT Scan machine, but they sell several to each hospital, then the hospital has to recommend unnecessary tests to compensate for the high cost of the machines.

I recall a famous physicist friend whose doctor told him he had mouth cancer with only six weeks to live and said he needed to "begin chemo and radiation immediately." The holistically aware physicist told him to forget it. (Not in those words.) He lived 12 more years well into his 70's and died peacefully in his sleep of a heart attack. This is not an unusual incident, but these stories seldom get published. The fear tactics used by doctors are completely unnecessary, but they work. Patients spend thousands of dollars for a so-called "cure" that breaks down their whole immune system. In far too many cases, the cancer returns after three to five years and the patient has to start treatment again. When the cancer returns, their immune system is so weakened, they die from the prescribed second or third round of treatments.

Over the years, I've interviewed some of the most successful alternative doctors in the world and learned that cancer is a systemic disease that requires eliminating toxins. Cutting or burning it out of a specific part of the body often doesn't do any good. Cutting into cancer more often than not causes the cells to spread throughout the system and chemo and radiation destroys the immune system.

Cancer is an imbalance that generally starts in the digestive system and the liver, that delivers the toxins to the most vulnerable parts of the body. Tumors are the body's own immune system creating a membrane to contain the toxins. Tumors can often be reduced by eliminating the poisons through diet, detoxing and utilizing various regimes of herbs, enzymes, oxygen, sound, light and chelation therapies, many of which are not allowed in America. However, there are dedicated physicians who use these methods because they don't want to rely on what they call the "Cut, Burn and Poison" procedures commonly accepted. They are doctors with a conscience - true healers who are willing to risk their own lives to heal their patients.

We simply can not trust the AMA and FDA to protect our food and health industries. They are overpowered by corporate giants who have the money and influence to pressure legislators, doctors and scientists to create biased research. They also keep a staff of public relations agents who make sure that the general public does not learn the truth about how they manufacture their products or the damage the additives used in processing are causing serious disease and even death. They have no conscience about the suffering and deaths they are causing. In actuality, there is little difference between these corporations and mass murderers, yet no one is saying this out loud and with the state of our current legislators, nothing is being done to stop them.

Every citizen of America should have the right to choose how to heal their body, but with this frightful dominance of the allopathic/chemical industrial complex, the power they have over Congress and the Senate and every medical association in the country, they do everything they can from allowing that to happen. With the billions of dollars demanded by Big Pharma in collusion with the allopathic medial profession and insurance companies, it's obvious that we need a medical revolution

CHAPTER 3

DR. MAX GERSON

IN THE 1930'S, A BRILLIANT German doctor named Max Gerson was the only doctor in the world curing tuberculosis. Around that time, Nobel Prize winner, Albert Schweitzer's wife came down with TB. They had traveled all over the world to find a cure and finally found their way to Dr. Gerson in Germany who was able to heal her.

Max was the only doctor who had taken the time to test how every food reacted in the body and he discovered that a vegetarian diet was the most healing.

Schweitzer was so impressed with Dr. Gerson's results, he invited him to testify before the US Congress. Understanding the risk of toxic food additives, Gerson explained to congress that if Americans would remove canned and frozen foods out of their diet, they would eradicate 80% of all disease - including cancer. The result was that the canned and frozen food industry immediately vilified him. Despite their ire, Max set up a clinic in California where he regularly cured cancer without chemo and radiation. However, it wasn't long before our government chased him out of the country forcing him to relocate his clinic in Mexico.

In the late 80's, I was invited to attended a lecture by Dr. Gerson's then 80-year-old daughter Charlotte. She explained how cancer is treated in their clinic, and the examples of overall healing they were able to accomplish with her father's dietary protocols. One of the most enlightening things she shared was that the emotions play a significant role in the development of the disease. "When a couple comes to our clinic, we refuse to take them unless they both go into counseling. There's always one person who gets the cancer and the other that gives it. If they don't agree to counseling, we won't take them as patients."

In addition to the vegetarian diet, she also mentioned that the first two things eliminated out of the diet are coffee and chocolate, which are highly acid forming foods. It's now recognized that cancer grows more readily in a highly acidic environment.

At the end of her talk, there were six former patients who had been healed at the Gerson clinic. Each of them said when they checked in, they didn't just have cancer, they had 4 or 5 other diseases such as heart trouble, diabetes, arthritis, digestive problems, etc. When they were released, all of their health problems were completely gone. Charlotte Gerson readily admitted there are some cases that do not get healed, but it is usually when the patient waits until they have gone through surgery, chemo and radiation and are on the verge of death before coming to the clinic.

At the end of the lecture, a man in the audience snarled at Charlotte, "If your father was so brilliant at healing, why isn't he alive today?" She answered, "Someone working in our clinic cafeteria poisoned my father's food. He died and there was never a formal investigation to identify the killer."

Charlotte Gerson is still thriving with good health today and is well into her 90's. There are many, many alternative doctors who are successfully healing cancer. I recommend, Barry Lynes book, *The Healing of Cancer,* written in 1989. He further explains the corruption of the industry and lists many of the well known doctors and methods of that period.

CHAPTER 4

AVOIDING BREAST CANCER

BECAUSE BREAST CANCER IS GETTING so much attention in the press, mostly from a profiteering perspective, I've chosen to specifically address this serious issue. Currently, one in 36 women will have breast cancer and it's second only to lung cancer in the leading cause of death. It's being reported that breast cancer has been declining since 1989 due to women cutting back in the use of female hormones. I am not convinced. Statistics are often manipulated or reported inaccurately to protect corporate interests.

It's actually surprising that the medical profession has admitted the link between hormones and breast cancer at all. The connection finally became so obvious, it could no longer be hidden. Only recently has it been reported that anyone who consumes large amounts of meat is more likely to develop cancer, however they do not mention the hormones added to meat and dairy as being the toxic link. The livestock industries obviously do not want to be implicated. The result is that those pertinent facts are not reported by the mainstream media.

It makes sense that if cattle or livestock are getting hormones to fatten quickly for market, those hormones would be the cause of most breast and uterine cancers - in addition to causing obesity. The hormone balance in humans and animals is delicate and can be easily altered by injecting foreign hormones or various chemicals, pesticides and pharmaceuticals. This is being proven daily by young boys and adult men who are now developing breasts and breast cancer. The same sex mating of birds and other animals has been attributed to the hormone damaging pesticides and herbicides discovered in our lakes, rivers and streams. Meddling with hormones by using pharmaceuticals that alter the natural hormonal balance is truly risking the reproductive systems of all living things. There is no hard research into the unknown long-term affects on our DNA and the development of future generations.

The good news is that women who are vegetarian have a significantly lower rate of cancer and woman who follow a Vegan diet have a dramatic 47% decrease in female specific cancers. That should be enough to convince any woman to avoid meat and dairy raised with hormones. If you do want to eat meat occasionally and want to be proactive in preventing your possible breast cancer, it's better to select meats and dairy raised on hormone-free farms where the animals are not fed genetically modified corn and where they are allowed to roam eating the grasses and wild herbs that have been their natural dietary heritage. There are wild grasses and weeds consumed by animals that provide important nutrition that have yet to be researched.

CHAPTER 5

PESTICIDES

~~~

IT HAS BEEN ABSOLUTELY PROVEN that Round-up and other pesticides using neonicotinoids, and imidacloprids are killing pollinators and are causing cancer, disease and the death of millions of humans, insect and animal species. Farmers around the world are experiencing major deaths among butterflies, bees and bats that are vital to our own survival. Without their gifts of pollination, most flowers and many vegetables can not produce - and human beings can not survive. Too little is being done to stop the use of these expensive pesticides that have been created by chemical companies like Monsanto, Archer Daniels Midland and others who control the agri-business industry that dominates both farming and the marketplace.

Some years ago, I was hired to write the copy for a pesticide company. To gain a clear understanding of how the company's product worked, I called the president who proudly explained that his poison killed insects by crystallizing their stomachs from the inside out. The millions of antacid commercials immediately leapt to my mind. I intuitively knew that if insects were being crystalized, our own digestive systems were being damaged by these harmful pesticides that are used daily by the agri-business industry.

As explained by Rudolph Steiner, the father of Bio-Dynamic gardening, every insect and animal on this earth - all life forms are vital to our own lives in ways that we have yet to completely understand. They are a part of the mysterious and magical chain of life. Being a head of his time, Steiner's theories are being proven daily by the Bio-Dynamic farmers who are using his organic methods and seeing the results. There is no denying that crops grown in soil being nurtured and fed properly, without harmful pesticides and herbicides are more healthful and delicious.

More and more of us are understanding how vitally important it is for people to eat, organically grown, pesticide-free, locally grown food that provides ultimate life force. The live enzymes provided by soil free of harmful additives are the foundation for creating our energy and overall health. Anything less is the path to disease.

CHAPTER 6

The Whole Truth About Tobacco

~~~~~

MANY YEARS AGO, I SMOKED only on the weekends when I was drinking and socializing. If I tried to smoke during the week when I wasn't drinking, it made me dizzy. The alcohol was obviously deadening my nervous system enough to allow me to poison myself. Then one day, I heard someone say, "When you inhale a cigarette, all of the oxygen is cut off to every organ of the body." It scared me so much, I quit. I just couldn't allow myself to continue doing something that was so harmful.

Most of us have no idea what is contained in tobacco or what's involved in the growing process. The following information came directly from the son of a flu-cured tobacco farmer in South Georgia who had worked on his father's farm and was eager to tell me how poisonous the crops were.

"In early December, the tobacco beds are prepared in the most fertile part of the field. Once the small plants are put in the soil, plastic is laid over the beds that are set a foot off the ground to protect them from freezing. After laying the plastic, to prevent weeds, the plants are regularly fumigated with poisons through a plastic pipe from the outside. Before these tender plants are pulled from these beds to be transplanted in the larger fields, they are fumigated and poisoned at least 6 to 8 more times to kill diseases, insects, and worms. Once transplanted to the larger fields, at the end of each row, to prevent root disease, the planter is refilled with water containing a toxic powder and the plants get watered with this poisonous water over, and over, again.

Suckers are the little stems that grow between the stalk and the leaf. They have to be cut off with a knife or they steal growth from the leaves. Tobacco has a flower that buds out at the top of the plant. It also has to be cut so that the leaves will grow large and healthy. Then, to keep the tops and suckers from growing back, the tobacco plants are sprayed with other chemicals that are mixed in the water.

Tobacco worms grow two to four inches long and are as big around as a man's finger. If the tobacco is not sprayed at least once a week, specifically for the worms, they eat the larger, more profitable leaves. As the plant ripens, flu cured tobacco is gathered by taking leaves from the bottom of the plant. The leaves are then put into barns to cure (or cook) for a week at a low temperature. There is no way that the poisons are not baked in. No one ever pulls the worms off that escape being killed and when the tobacco leaves spill on the floor, they are simply swept up with the rest of the dirt and bugs and put back into the bins.

Several different manufacturers produce the various chemical poisons used on tobacco. They vary widely from area to area, and often from farm to farm, but the result is the same, tobacco is sprayed with chemical poisons at least two dozen times or more, before harvest."

This gentleman's story helps you understand why smoking, along with second-hand smoke is so dangerous. The fumes from the toxins applied in the field are a major reason why hospitals are full of tobacco related cancers, COPD, emphysema, lung, throat and breathing problems.

During congressional discussions over tobacco legislation, not one word is ever mentioned about the growth poisons and pesticides utilized in the manufacturing process. To ensure this information is not revealed, industry tobacco farmers and chemical pesticide manufacturers maintain their control by donating huge amounts of money to political campaigns and offer luxurious perks to the legislators who support them.

With this first hand knowledge, in addition to knowing that with every puff of a cigarette, the oxygen is cut off from your organs and spinal cord, I hope this direct information will inspire anyone who smokes to consider how much damage they are doing to their bodies and the consequences they will suffer.

CHAPTER 7

ALCOHOL RELATED CANCERS

HISTORICALLY, THE DRINKING OF ALCOHOL has been so socially acceptable that it has become society's beloved escape. It stylishly swallows everyone into a state of total denial that causes most of us to overlook all of it's physical and mental health destroying properties. Hangovers and vomiting are minor symptom compared to what alcohol does to your overall system. The slurred speech, the impairment of coordination and balance are those attributes that we are all aware but, we don't recognize them as serious signals that are all too often overlooked or viewed as being amusing. They aren't amusing at all, they are the body's warnings that you're consuming a toxic substance that like cigarettes, will slowly cause eventual disease and death. Even moderate drinking combined with cigarettes dramatically increases the risk of upper respiratory and colon cancers, especially in women.

Alcohol is a highly toxic substance that facilitates emotional denial, millions of car accidents, innumerable diseases and ruined lives. It's clearly one of the toxins that should be avoided when trying to sustain a healthy, productive life.

The fact seldom mentioned is that regular drinkers age much faster than those who do not imbibe or who rarely drink. It shows in their face with wrinkles, deep lines, sagging skin and reddish coloring. All of these are indications of the breakdown of bodily tissue, as is the facial bloating and enlarged red nose which indicates high levels of alcohol toxicity. Unfortunately, most doctors today are not trained to look at these signs as the beginning of disease.

Placing the body in a state of endangerment at every level, drinkers tend to have more arthritis, rheumatism, joint stiffness and eventual calcification of the overall body. Pancreatitis, cirrhosis of the liver, hypoglycemia and serious complications for diabetics occur with heavy drinkers, as well as sexual dysfunction and critical birth defects. In addition to malnutrition and numbness of the hands and feet, it causes vulnerability of the lungs leading to colds, bacterial infections and pneumonia.

Women alcohol drinkers are more likely to develop breast cancer and heavy drinkers among both sexes increase their risk of mouth, throat and esophageal cancers.

Drinking causes damage to the nervous system and affects the brain by shrinking the lobes eventually causing dementia. The heart is also greatly affected by alcohol in that it causes irregular heartbeat, high blood pressure, heart attack and stroke.

Alcohol damages the whole digestive system and the symptoms are seldom recognized as being related to alcohol. Starting in the mouth, alcohol causes gum disease, tooth decay and tooth loss. In the digestive tract it can be the cause of ulcers, heartburn, swollen stomach, indigestion, inflammation of the stomach lining and irritation to the colon. This is in addition to vomiting, hemorrhoids and diarrhea. The list goes on and on.

As adults, we need to be less naive about the pleasant escape provided by alcohol. With the heavy drinking socially accepted among teenagers in America today, they need to be better informed as to the dangerous patterns they're creating which often pave their way to alcohol addiction.

CHAPTER 8

SUGAR AND THE LOSS OF WILL

THE MESSAGE OF THIS BOOK would be incomplete without addressing sugar, which is one of the greatest health enemies of our time. Sugar causes more health problems than cigarettes, cocaine, marijuana, heroin, alcohol, or any other addictive substance, but because it kills slowly, it's overlooked.

Sugar leaches vital minerals and enzymes that are the necessary catalysts in the digestion process that carry oxygen and nourishment to the cells and brain.

Sugar addictions begin at birth when we put honey as a sweetener in the baby's bottle to make it emulate the natural sweetness of mother's milk. It continues with the peanut butter and jelly sandwiches packed in school lunches and when we bribe our children to eat with the promise of dessert. It's mindlessly supported in nursery school with cookie breaks. It's carried on in high school, college and offices across America where snack machines and school cafeterias are controlled by the sugar and soft drink industry. Cookies and sweets are the mainstay at neighborhood gatherings and church socials.

Can any of us forget Sesame Street's "Cookie Monster. It's literally impossible to escape America's addiction to sweets.

Inordinate cravings for quick, energy producing foods are often due to the depletion of the nutrients in our soils. We are simply not getting the nutrition in corporately grown foods to support our physical and mental health, so we often grab the quickest energy boost we can find. It's easy to substitute some of the many delicious fruits and nuts sold in markets, but we often don't make those choices.

The most frustrating thing about sugar is that it is now added to everything, even cigarettes. Sweet sells! Unless otherwise stated, practically everything packaged or processed in any way has sugar added and, the sugar industry does an impeccable job of marketing. Conversely, healthy, natural products such as fruit and nuts are seldom made available as a wholesome alternative.

Too much sugar in the diet is responsible for diabetes, arthritis, hair loss, obesity, rheumatism, low blood sugar, skin disorders, callouses and a host of other so-called chronic diseases. It's often the source of headaches, cramps, back and muscle aches, yet is usually overlooked as a cause.

Sugar processing is similar to cocaine. The cocoa leaf by itself is chewed by natives to give them a boost of energy while planting and harvesting in the mountainous fields in Peru. It's a fairly harmless plant if used only occasionally, but if chewed daily, it causes rotting teeth and other health complications. In the refining process, like sugarcane, coca leaves are cooked and bleached resulting in the white powder that becomes highly addictive due to the loss of natural minerals in the plant. Like cocaine, sugar leaches the body's store of minerals needed in the digestive process. That loss of minerals is what produces the constant craving. What people don't realize is that sugar is 8 times more addictive than cocaine and causes the death of over 600,000 people yearly.

The delicious combination of chocolate and sugar sets up an unnatural craving that haunts us all of our lives. Like smoking and taking drugs, sugar causes a loss of will. It literally creates weakened human beings. How many of us have friends who are diabetics and despite the fact they know sugar is killing them, they will endure having their legs amputated rather than stop eating sugar and chocolate. If you are a coffee or tea drinker, unless you are drinking your coffee black, don't think you are just addicted to the caffeine, you're probably addicted to the sugar fix as well. Recognizing these sugar addictions, you begin to understand why people need to have their caffeine/sugar fix in the morning and throughout the day to keep them going.

The global addiction to sugar is so widely accepted, it's like there's a contest to see who can dream up the richest, most decadent combinations. Some of us remember the days when our taste buds were satisfied with the simple ice cream selections of vanilla, chocolate and strawberry. We were thrilled to eat Neapolitan that was a combination of the three flavors. Now, we have chocolate desserts, ice cream sundaes and float combinations called Chocolate Overdose, Better Than Sex, Cake Dough, Chocolate Marshmallow Caramel

Fudge, Chocolate Carmel Peanut Butter, etc. etc. The more sickening sweet combinations the better. The ungodly combinations go on ad nauseam.

Now there's chocolate cereals, chocolate bubble gum, and even chocolate served in the morning on toast. These chocolate/sugar infusions initiate the path to diabetes, especially for children. Once your tongue gets used to such an overload of sugary tastes, simple tastes become boring. You begin wanting sugar in every thing you eat. In canned and packaged foods, that's exactly what you're getting. Our taste buds have become so jaded - we may as well just take the chocolate and inject it directly in our veins. They don't call it "Devils Food" for nothing.

Without eliminating sugar from the diet, it's difficult to discern the difference in how you can think and feel. When Madison Ave. is drumming at you through television and advertising to eat or drink, this or that, it's easy to fall prey to their temptations. Instead of eating candy bars and other junk foods with sugar added, it takes continuing willpower to make the wise decision to substitute fruit and nuts or even fresh vegetables for our cravings.

CHAPTER 9

Aspartame

~~~~~

IN ATLANTA, IN THE EARLY 90's, I had a talk show called Health Frontiers. One of my guests was Betty Martini, founder of Mission Possible International. This amazing woman has single handedly educated millions of people worldwide as to the dangers of aspartame.

Since then, every time I see someone order a diet coke, I want to shout Stop, Don't Drink That! It will eventually cause a serious health problem!

When I try to tell women about aspartame, they just ignore me or think I'm being overly paranoid. The truth is that the FDA has received more complaints about aspartame than any other product besides MSG. Because it has been proven to be a neurotoxin, doctors from all over the nation have instigated legislation to have Aspartame removed from the market, but nothing has been done. More attentive to the dangers of chemical additives than the FDA, the European Union has in fact outlawed aspartame in infants and children's products.

Aspartame contains three highly toxic substances, aspartic acid, methanol and in temperatures over 86, formaldehyde.

Formaldehyde is used in embalming. Think about how many times cases of diet drinks sit in trucks, warehouses or in front of gas stations where temperatures reach the 90's?

Manufactured by Monsanto, Aspartame is a sweetener found in almost everything under the camouflaged names of Equal, NutraSweet, Spoonful, Benevia, NatraTaste, Truvia, etc. It's even in adult and children's vitamins, children's cookies, fast food treats and in many packaged and frozen foods.

Many years ago, Senator Howard Metzenbaum told Dr. Kessler of the FDA, that aspartame should never have been approved. Tests conducted in the 1940's by the American Bottling Association absolutely proved that aspartame caused brain tumors in mice and rats, in addition to seizures in five of seven primates. It should never been permitted.

In his book *Excitotoxins: The Taste That Kills,* Neurologist Russell L. Blaylock, says,"the reactions to aspartame are not allergic in nature, but are as toxic as arsenic and cyanide. Aspartame is a dangerous neurotoxin and a significant carcinogen for many organs. It should be avoided at all cost. The ingredients in aspartame literally stimulate the neurons to death causing brain damage of varying degrees." Blaylock explains that, "Aspartic acid is known to be an excitotoxin lowering the seizure threshold, especially under hypoglycemic conditions. When mixed with other excitotoxins such as MSG, it greatly increases the likelihood of adverse reactions."

Emory University Pediatric Professor, Dr. Louis Elsas, testified before Congress identifying aspartame as a deadly neurotoxin and teratogin that triggers birth defects. He cited cases of women who were heavy diet coke drinkers having as many as seven miscarriages.

Many, many people suffer from aspartame problems their doctors can't identify or make a connection. That is, until the patient stops drinking diet cokes or eating products with NutraSweet. Then their symptoms disappear, unless it's too late and serious disease has already begun.

Dave Reitz, suffered joint pain that was so unbearable, it kept him in a Jacuzzi for years. His doctors never associated his problems with aspartame. On the Internet, he discovered the FDA report of 92 documented symptoms including joint pain, coma, seizures and death. After stopping aspartame, his pain disappeared. He later established his web site, dorway.com relaying personal experiences and documented physician's research, including the FDA files. He says,"I want to give back to the Internet what the Internet gave back to me - my life."

Due to the increase in unexplainable seizures among airline pilots, most airlines will not allow their pilots to drink diet drinks. In May of 1992, due to the increased possibility of seizures, vertigo and vision loss, *Flying Safety,* the journal of the U.S. Air Force warned all pilots to avoid aspartame.

Endocrinologist, Dr. H. J Roberts, in his book, *Aspartame Disease: The Ignored Epidemic,* calls Aspartame Disease a worldwide epidemic causing seizures, stroke, MS, heart failure, blindness, liver problems, lupus, mental confusion, disorientation, and numerous other cardiac and neurological disorders. Having studied Alzheimer's for 30 years, Roberts wrote a 700-page Pulitzer Prize winning research treatise stating that aspartame causes Alzheimer's. In conjunction with the research of many other doctors and activists, Dr. Roberts submitted his findings to the FDA and the US Congress, but no legislation has been passed to stop its use.

In the 1960's, despite Monsanto knowing Aspartame caused tumors, they set up a subsidiary called Searle Laboratories making Donald Rumsfeld President. It was Rumsfeld that manipulated it through the legislature getting it wrongfully legalized. Due to powerful lobbyists funded by Monsanto, Coca Cola and other diet food manufacturers, it still hasn't been taken out of the marketplace.

For years, Monsanto has continued to deny the research against aspartame. Removing all of their products from the market could be a bigger financial loss than tobacco. Knowing this, the corporation began buying up all of the Stevia farms they can acquire to eventually replace Aspartame. One of Coke's latest products has a combination of sugar and Stevia which is a harmless sweetener made from the root of a plant in the Chrysanthemum family. It's been found in health food stores as a sugar substitute for over 25 years. Stevia is calorie free, does not cause sugar highs, aids digestion and has been safely used in the Orient for years. Depending on the manufacturer, sometimes Stevia can have a bitter or strong after taste but is a healthy alternative.

CHAPTER 10

Fluoridation

Fluoride is another one of the most poisonous chemicals in our environment that our legislators have permitted it in our water systems since the 1940's. We consume it daily.

John Yiamouyiannis is recognized as an international authority on the biologic effects of Fluoride and has served as the Science Consultant on Fluoridation in the US and abroad. He explains that when chemical companies find themselves stuck with waste products, they often find ways to utilize them in the mainstream. Fluoride is an actual poisonous by-product of the aluminum and phosphate fertilizer industries. When scientists objected to the dumping of Fluoride into rivers and lakes, to justify it as safe, the fertilizer industry decided to add it to drinking water and it was quickly approved by our Congress.

According to Nobel Prize winner Dr. William Murphy, "Fluorides can cause dental mottling, skin eruptions, tongue sores, eczema, hives, gastritis, headache and muscle weakness. However, these hypersensitive reactions usually disappear promptly after discontinuation of the chemical. Fluoridation is responsible for the chronic poisoning of over 130 million Americans, a substantial number of which are suffering from arthritis. There are over 8 million American children who are so badly poisoned, their teeth are discolored and 2 million who suffer from allergic reactions. In 1997, Dr. Murphy contended there were 35,000 Americans who die from fluoridation each year and 100,000 who die from fluoridation-induced cancers. Those numbers have increased dramatically.

Fluoride is added to the public water system at the rate of about 1 to 3 parts per million. Yiamouyiannis says it is more poisonous than lead, just slightly less poisonous than arsenic, and has been used as a pesticide to control mice, rats and other small pests. As we are all aware, Fluoride has been promoted as retarding tooth decay, however there is no proof at all that it has been effective.

Yiamouyiannis quotes a spokesman from Procter and Gamble, the makers of Crest toothpaste acknowledging that a family-sized tube of Fluoride toothpaste "theoretically" contains enough Fluoride to kill a small child."

Says Yiamouyiannis, "While no one is going to die from drinking one glass of fluoridated water, just as no one will die from smoking one cigarette, it is the longer-term chronic effects of glass after glass of fluoridated water that takes its toll in human health and life."

In 1992, the Canadian Dental Association refused to condone the use of Fluoride for children less than three years old. Their research proved that it interferes with the proper formation of collagen and collagen-like proteins in the teeth during formative stages. Fluoridated water also lends to the breakdown of proteins that comprise the structural component for skin, ligaments, muscles, cartilage and bone.

The ability of Fluoride to transform normal cells into cancer cells was confirmed by Argonne National Laboratories, which also found that "Fluoride increases the cancer causing ability of other chemicals." Battelle Research Institute conducted a two-year study on rats and mice and found "an iron-clad link between Fluoride exposure and an extremely rare form of liver cancer in Fluoride treated male and female mice."

The Journal of the American Medical Association published three separate articles linking increased hip fracture rates to fluoridated areas. The New England Journal of Medicine found that Fluoride causes osteoporosis and bone fractures, prematurely wrinkled skin, arthritis, torn ligaments, genetic damage and increases in tumor growth at a rate of 25%. It has also been strongly linked as one of the causes of Attention Deficit Disorder, birth defects and the lowering of intelligence.

The proof of Fluoride related problems is frightening and yet, our local officials are not acting on these disturbing facts because they are purposely kept in the dark as to the truth. Until the public is made aware and makes demands to omit the use of this highly toxic substance, it's wise to avoid fluoridated water for drinking or cooking by obtaining pure spring or purified water, **preferably not in plastic bottles.**

CHAPTER 11

Avoiding Microwaved Foods - Even for Coffee & Tea

With the statistics of cancer on a continual rise, we need to put microwaves high on the list of cancer causing agents.

Today, both singles and families eat out much more than in the past and most restaurant foods are heated with microwave ovens - especially fast food chains. Toaster ovens really are much safer and healthier than microwaves and take only a few minutes longer to warm or even bake food, but in most homes, they have been cast aside.

Some years ago, I took a Windjammer sailing cruise and one of my wonderful shipmates was a physicist from Georgia Tech. At night, we would all sit on deck talking, laughing and looking at the stars. One evening, the subject of microwave ovens came up and he warned us that microwaved foods were absolutely detrimental to human health. I heeded his advice and have never owned one. Later, I came across an extremely important bit of research that substantiated the physicist's advice.

Working with Bernard H. Blanc of the Swiss Federal Institute of Technology and the University Institute for Biochemistry, Hans Ulrich Hertel was one of the first scientists recognized for conducting and personally participating in a quality study on the degenerative effects of microwaved nutrients on food, human blood and the overall physiology of humans.

The research proved conclusively that microwaved foods had their nutrients changed so significantly, they altered blood hemoglobin causing deterioration to human biological systems. In addition to the reduced hemoglobin, the research cited a decrease in all cholesterol values, particularly altering the value and ratio between the HDL (good cholesterol) and LDL (bad cholesterol).

In 1991, Hertel and his colleague, a Lausanne University professor published a research paper indicating that food cooked in microwave ovens could pose a greater health risk than foods cooked by conventional means. This led Hertel to the conclusion that the energies may indeed be passed along to humans when they consume microwaved food.

An article appeared in issue #19 of *The Swiss Journal* in which Franz Weber clearly stated that the consumption of food cooked in microwave ovens had cancer-type effects on the blood. They later published the actual research paper.

On August 7, 1992, the Swiss Association of Manufacturers and Suppliers of Household Appliances took action against Hertel in Berne's Commercial Court charging that the applicants research was "worthless and his findings untenable." As often happens, Hertel was quickly quieted with a gag order by the Swiss Association of Dealers of Electroapparatuses for Households and Industry, known as the FEA.

However, in 1998 that decision was reversed. In a judgment delivered at Strasbourg on August 25, 1998, in the case of Hertel v. Switzerland, the European Court of Human Rights held that there had been a violation of Hertel's rights in the 1993 decision. The Court ruled that the "gag order" issued by the Swiss courts against Hertel was contrary to the right to freedom of expression. In addition, Switzerland was sentenced to pay compensation of F40,000 to cover legal costs and expenses. This decision put an end to judicial censorship of persons drawing attention to the health hazards of certain products.

The Europeans have much better control over their food industry than our FDA. They have outlawed GMO's, American meats grown with hormones and they avoid the use of harmful pesticides. I tend to trust their research more because it is not funded by the manufacturers of the harmful products themselves.

CHAPTER 12

TOXIC INGREDIENTS

LIKE FLUORIDE AND ASPARTAME, THERE are so many additives and preservatives added to our foods, that if given in large doses are poison. Repeated day after day, those small doses eventually cause serious disease. It is our tendency to view allergic reactions as less threatening, but continual irritation of the immune system by allergens can eventually cause serious illness and chronic disease.

All of us are bombarded with toxins in our daily lives which includes harmful pesticides like Round-Up and hormones like rBGH and other growth factors given to livestock to fatten them quickly for market. In the process, our delicate hormonal systems are thrown out of balance. As mentioned earlier, too few of us have made the connection that these hormones could be the major cause of obesity in America today. It seems like common sense that if we are imbibing these fattening hormones through our meat and dairy products, they are being absorbed in the digestion process and we too will fatten quickly. Our bodies are not meant to handle foreign hormones, which are the unspoken cause of breast, uterine, prostrate and other forms of cancer.

Under the over-simplified, cryptic term GMO or Genetically Modified Organism, it is highly disturbing to learn the actual meaning of genetically modified. It means that food manufacturers are using animal and insect genes to create longer shelf life. For example, firefly genes are spliced into tomatoes to induce longer shelf life and it was recently revealed that hot dogs contain human DNA. There is no long-term testing taking place to determine what future affects this will have on the human race. Often called Frankinfoods, I call them Demon Foods. Only a demonic mind would consider altering the DNA of the human race without knowing the result. Combining genes from different species is a frightening gamble we should not be taking. The truth is that we have been reduced to lab rats in the hands of Agri-business giants.

Cancer and most diseases start in the digestive system - particularly the liver which is our most important digestive organ that removes toxins from the body. The French know about keeping the liver healthy, but you will never hear an American doctor telling you to do a liver cleanse, to detox the body or to even consider the health of your liver. Allopathic doctors are not trained to preserve organs. It will never come up in the conversation.

Let us not overlook foods being radiated. Unless locally grown, most of our foods and spices are being nuked, especially when imported from foreign countries. This means that most transported foods have traces of radiation. Like microwave ovens, radiating foods kills off vital enzymes crucial to the digestive process.

Most people ignore the warning signs of indigestion, gas or other digestive problems; they don't make the connection to the foods they're consuming. Think about all of the Tums, anti-acids, and prescriptions to aid digestion administered by doctors. Stress is not the only cause.

The Creator did a wonderful job of balancing nature and the miraculous workings of the human body. Agri-business scientists think they can do it better by radiating, adding hormones and splicing genes from other beings. There are too few of us doing anything about it, because we are not told the whole truth about what is being done to our foods.

Since being domesticated, animals are now suffering from indigestion, allergies and are dying from the diseases that modern man continually succumb. The recent increase of yearly vaccines and the use of poisons to deter fleas is also contributing to the organ diseases of domesticated pets. Birds, insects and animals living in the wild are dying from environmental poisons which is further evidence of the toxins to which we are all exposed.

CHAPTER 13

MSG

MSG, Monosodium Glutamate originated from a Japanese scientist who isolated it from Kombu, a healthy, flavorful seaweed used in Japanese cooking. It was found to enhance the quality of taste by suppressing the bitterness, sourness and the tinny taste of canned foods. However, MSG is actually one of the most poisonous additives we have in our foods.

According to Dr. George R. Schwartz, author of, *In Bad Taste: The MSG Syndrome,* MSG is a perfect example of a poison we've been getting in our foods for over 50 years. He says, "MSG is not just an allergen - it is a poison that is absolutely detrimental to everyone at varying doses."

Schwartz cites a case history of a hospitalized young woman with an undetermined neurologic ailment. She had previously seen several neurologists, none of whom were able to help her. Existing only on intravenous feeding, her weight fell to 77 pounds and she was continuing to deteriorate.

The woman happened to catch a radio interview with Dr. Schwartz and immediately contacted him. Her seriously poor health turned out to be a severe MSG reaction. Every time she had shown improvement, the nurses gave her the typical clear broth containing MSG that is served in all hospitals, and her condition would worsen. She's fine now as long as she stays away from MSG which is commonly used in most canned and packaged foods. The Boullion and Jello fed to people in hospitals are both processed with MSG, however doctors and nurses are not educated as to the toxins in foods. That's one of the reasons it makes sense to recuperate at home, instead of in a hospital.

While this young woman's degree of sensitivity may be unusual, she represents a growing percentage of people who react violently to low doses of MSG that others seem to tolerate, or they simply don't connect the headache or other symptoms they suffer after eating MSG as being related. Her case is a perfect example of what can happen as the chemical keeps accumulating in our bodies.

MSG is an excitatory neurotransmitter which causes the nerve cells to discharge an electrical impulse. That's the basis of its use as a flavor enhancer. It electrically excites the nerves that support the tasting process. But, that is also the basis for most of its many side effects. The most common negative reaction to MSG is a headache, but it can also cause a dangerous, irregular heart beat; difficulty in concentration; extreme mood swings such as depression, anger, paranoia, balance problems, and in some severe cases, convulsions or suicide.

In children, MSG and other preservatives over stimulate the brain and can result in hyperactivity, sleep disturbances, convulsions, angry outbursts, screaming, learning difficulties and can affect digestion by causing stomach cramps and diarrhea. It can also irritate the esophagus causing acid reflux, heartburn, asthma, throat swelling, acid reflux, heartburn, frequent urination, incontinence and in some men and prostate disorders. It never occurs to most doctors that MSG may be the cause of these problems because they are kept ill informed and do not have the time to re-educate themselves.

By eating out in restaurants or consuming a continual diet of canned and processed foods, Schwartz says we are continuing to receive additional doses all day. "Those people who think they aren't bothered by MSG are reacting, whether they recognize it or not. Physiologically, at the cellular level, body processes are being disturbed in subtle ways." Often, people who react with headaches, like Schwartz himself, do not make the connection between what they are eating and the problems that ensue. "One patient had diarrhea for over 20 years, until we discovered the cause. Another had numbness in the jaw as their primary symptom. Whatever the symptom, with subsequent exposure to MSG, they will exhibit the same symptom again and again."

Schwartz explains that American industry is too heavily invested in MSG to ever give it up voluntarily. "Nothing short of sweeping legislation could turn it around now and that isn't likely. Despite the large numbers of written complaints and reports of serious reactions (and even deaths) from physicians and researchers, the pro-MSG industry continues to claim the allergies are a myth. As a toxicologist, I assure you, this if far from the truth."

In the late 1960's, MSG was removed from baby food, but it is now difficult to find any processed food that doesn't contain MSG, which is also found under the names of; Monopotassium Glutamate, Glutamate, Glutamic Acid, Gelatin, Hydrolyzed Vegetable Protein, Hydrolyzed Plant Protein, Autolyzed Plant Protein, Sodium Caseinate, Calcium Caseinate, Textured Protein Yeast Extract, Yeast food or nutrient and Autolyzed yeast.

Bacon, ham, salami and various sausages contain MSG, in addition to food dyes, all of which are highly toxic. The same is true for most chips.

Ice cream is a perfect example of a food we don't expect to contain harmful preservatives. In most ice creams manufactured by large corporations, you will find a number of unpronounceable ingredients. If you can't pronounce them, if they contain any kind of food coloring, or if the label says anything but milk, cream, sugar or flavoring; put it back in the freezer and find another one that's healthier. Publix makes an organic alternative with just a few ingredients.

As home makers, we have to take responsibility for preserving our own and our family's health by making educated choices in the marketplace. It's important to read labels and to avoid packaged, processed and frozen foods. Many home makers and TV Chefs try to gain popularity by suggesting quick cooking time and convenience. They promote greens and vegetables that are cleaned, chopped and sold in plastic bags. Those plastic bags and saran wrappings exude chemicals that are highly toxic to the body. In addition they can contain bacteria that cause such diseases as salmonella, E.coli, and Listeria. They should be avoided in favor of fresh unpackaged vegetables.

* Any kind of plastic container expels harmful gases. In the case of melons, it's best to remove the saran wrap and use wax paper to cover them, or cut them up and store them in a glass container, not plastic!

CHAPTER 14

FOOD COLORING

THE FDA HAS ALREADY RECOGNIZED food colorings as poisons that cause cancerous tumors yet, they still have not been removed from the marketplace. This is in spite of the fact, that it has been known for many years that both food dyes and food additives like MSG cause hyperactivity in children.

When I see those highly decorated cakes and cupcakes in bakeries with their frightfully unnatural pigments, especially the vivid blue, all I see is illness. Don't let these exotic colors lure you; they are poisonous to your children.

* That scary Brilliant Blue #1 is known to cause kidney tumors in rats. In addition to bake goods, it is found in the new funky, blue colored beverages, dessert powders, candies, cereals and even over-the-counter drugs and pharmaceutical prescriptions.

* Blue dye #2 causes brain tumors and is found in both human and dog food.

* Red #2 also causes tumors in bladder and other organs. It's used in the coloration of oranges. (If you are sensitive, it accounts for the bitterness you taste when it gets on your fingers in the process of peeling.)

* Red dye #3 is a thyroid carcinogen used in maraschino cherries. It's also found in sausage casings, oral medications, frostings and candies.

* Red dye #40 which is the most-widely used, is suspected to cause immune system tumors. It also causes allergic reactions and is found in colas, bakery goods, dessert powders, candies, cereals, many canned foods, cosmetics and medicines.

* Green dye #3 causes bladder and testes tumors in male rats and is found in candies, sodas, ice cream, sorbet, medicines, lip stick, cosmetics and other personal care products.

* Yellow #5 can also cause severe allergic reactions. It's used in pet foods, colorful bakery goods, sodas, dessert powders, candies, cereals, gelatin, desserts, and many other foods, as well as pharmaceutical meds and cosmetics.

* Yellow Dye #6 causes severe allergic reactions, in addition to adrenal tumors in animals. It's also found in colored bakery goods, cereals, sodas, dessert powders, candies, gelatin desserts, sausage, cosmetics, and drugs.

Most of these food dyes are labeled so you can identify them. If you start reading labels, you will be surprised to see that hundreds of foods and drugs contain these known poisonous substances. Knowing that food dyes and preservatives are as toxic as they are, its time we started asking pharmaceutical companies to stop using these substances in their medications.

For mothers who are baking cakes, cupcakes and colorful frostings, it's easy to substitute, strawberry, raspberry jams or jellies for red or pink - or even cranberry juice. Any kind of liquid chlorophyll product can be used for the green color; there's enough sugar in baked goods, the kids will never notice the difference. Blueberry and grape juice are good options for blue and purple. You can use your imagination to create other safe substitutes. The idea is to avoid giving these poisons to your children.

It has just been announced that due to the growing complaints about the food dyes and other toxic preservatives in our foods, some of the cereal companies have stopped using food dyes.

CHAPTER 15

WHEAT & GLUTEN

~~~

AFTER THOUSANDS OF YEARS OF being the mainstay of the human diet, and spending decades where most of us were raised on some kind of lunch sandwich, it's a frustrating challenge to eliminate bread from our diet. However, we are now being confronted with information that has emerged proving that wheat and gluten can be harmful to the body, especially for those who suffer celiac disease.

Gluten is everywhere. Barley, wheat, oats, rye and spelt all contain gluten. Most people know how addictive sugar is, but they don't realize that gluten is just as addictive. It causes ongoing craving - especially if you are gluten sensitive.

Unfortunately, continual bombardment of gluten in the immune system can lead to degeneration of the intestinal wall causing nutrient deficiencies. It's the source of various digestive issues, anemia, fatigue, dementia and other serious diseases.

Many gluten sensitive people suffer from acute bloating, gas and digestive disorders, in addition to bone and joint pain - especially among seniors who suffer knee, foot and leg problems. Along with sugar, it has also been found to accelerate tremors and Parkinson's disease. The sticky protein solution produced by gluten known as gliaden is often interpreted by cells as bacteria causing the body to literally attack itself. This leads to the breakdown of the digestive walls, leaky bowl syndrome and sluggishness in the blood stream.

In non-celiac gluten sensitivity, there is no attack on the body's own tissues, however many people suffer the same symptoms of bloating, stomach pain, indigestion, gas, fatigue, diarrhea and acute pain in bones and joints.

There is a sizable body of research coming out of Europe indicating that the mercury derivative used to preserve Monsanto's Round-Up-Ready seeds is also contributing greatly to wheat allergies.

If you will pay attention to how you feel after eating bread, pasta or any kind of wheat starch, you will observe that you become drowsy, wanting to sleep and needing to drink something with caffeine to keep you going. The more you pay attention to how you feel after meals, the more aware you become of the foods that either energize or deplete your body, so you can begin increasing or avoiding them.

Rice or bean noodles found in Chinese markets are a tasty substitute for wheat pasta. In addition to suggesting gluten-free breads which often aren't very appetizing, more and more chefs are suggesting greens like romaine lettuce, kale or chard to contain sandwich items. It's lighter, healthier and very flavorful.

For gluten sensitive people, Dr. Dietrich Klinghardt, suggests using the acronym **BROWS** as a reminder for **Barley, Rye, Oats, Wheat and Spelt**, that are the flours to avoid.

CHAPTER 16

Dairy Products

TRYING TO TAKE DAIRY AWAY from Caucasians is like trying to remove mother's milk from a baby. All of us in America and Europe love our dairy. Whether it's familiar products such as butter, milk, cottage cheese, yogurt, sour cream and whip cream, or the more sophisticated European cheeses, dairy has been the foundation of almost every culture on the planet, with exception of people from Asia.

Humans are the only species that drink milk after infancy and are the only ones who drink the milk of other species, with the rare exception of the people of Northern Africa, where in countries like Eritrea, camel milk is used for digestive problems.

Dairy in general is not good for our health. It causes mucous in the body and produces a highly acidic climate creating a fertile ground for the development of cancer.

Milk advertisements will tell you it builds strong bones, but it does just the opposite, it increases osteoporosis. Like wheat, dairy products cause swelling in the joints that irritate arthritis and rheumatism. It's also known to accelerate pain and the length of healing time in broken bones and ligaments. Because dairy is mucous forming, it can cause sinus, hay fever, vaginal yeast and various allergies. Dairy is also the major cause of clogged arteries, heart disease and stroke.

Milk is extremely harmful if it comes from corporate farms where livestock is raised with antibiotics in their feed and given GMO's, rBGH and IGF-1 hormones to fatten them quickly for market. As explained earlier, using the cryptic term GMO, Genetically Modified Organisms, doesn't tell the whole story. It actually means that scientists are splicing the genes of insects and animals into our meats, fruits and vegetables. They're like mad scientists playing roulette with our gene pool and possibly altering the future of the human race. Unless otherwise notified on the labels, this is what happens in most large American dairy farms, that's why labeling laws are so important.

On Agri-business farms, cows are never allowed to eat their normal diet of pesticide-free grass and wild greens that aid them in their own healthy digestive processes. Instead, they are given high doses of antibiotics to combat the bacteria and diseases that occur because they are cruelly confined in small cages where they defecate on themselves. Their feed includes a chemical concoction of antibiotics, steroids, hormones, cottonseed, animal products, chicken manure, genetically modified corn, pesticides, fungicides and a host of other chemicals foreign to our systems. So-called milk from Agri-business giants, is not milk, it is a manufactured highly toxic facsimale in which many of the hormones, particularly IGD-1 is known to cause breast, colon and prostate cancer. All of these highly toxic and foreign substances become infused in the meats we eat and contribute to the development of various forms of cancer, obesity and allergies.

When rBGH growth hormone is given to fatten livestock quickly, it accelerates their metabolism which causes them to be hungry all of the time. They are then given meat to quell their hunger. Cows are vegetarians and do not have the enzymes to properly digest meat. This is the cause of Mad Cow Disease which has now crossed over into humans and is often diagnosed as Alzheimers.

In the late 90's, I interviewed a nurse in Highlands, NC who told me her father died of what doctors had diagnosed as Alzheimers. She said, "I don't know why, but I decided I wanted to do an autopsy. The results showed Mad Cow Disease, not Alzheimers - which leads me to believe that this may account for the increasing incidences of so-called Alzheimer's in younger and younger people."

In this unnatural process of fattening livestock quickly for market, the abnormal doses of growth hormones is not only causing breast cancer in women, it is causing young men to develop breasts. When this occurs, most families don't discuss this embarrassing situation, but today, it's happening with greater and greater frequency.

All dairy products sold in super markets are pasteurized and/or homogenized to kill the bacteria that increases due to the animals being caged and defecating on themselves.

This processing kills the natural, life-given proteins, vitamins and enzymes provided by raw milk from untainted cows that are allowed to graze naturally. The result is, you are drinking a manufactured substance that, instead of feeding your body, upsets your digestion. In addition, dairy products cause weight gain, particularly around the breast and stomach and are often the cause of vaginal yeast, which most allopathic doctors refuse to recognize. They would rather prescribe vaginal creams that do nothing to eradicate the cause of the problem.

After years of suffering from vaginal yeast and going through dozens and dozens of tubes of Monistat or other useless options, only after hearing a lecture by macrobiotic advocate, Mishio Kushi did I learn that dairy products cause vaginal yeast and fatty cysts in the breast and vaginal area. Dairy can also cause cysts in other parts of the body that often appear just under the skin.

In addition to decreasing the risk of heart attacks and strokes, eliminating dairy from the diet can bring about demonstrable weight loss, especially for women whose breast size increases in their aging years.

If you are a dairy eater, it's vitally important to buy organically raised dairy products or to buy European cheeses. Europe has much stronger dietary controls than America. Like Canada and New Zealand, they do not allow the use of deadly hormones.

CHAPTER 17

COSMETIC TOXINS

※

ALL OF US, AT ONE time or another, have looked at the labels on various cosmetic items and shook our heads wondering what the heck all of those ingredients are that you can barely read, let alone pronounce. I'm sure you have noticed that the print gets smaller and smaller every year.

Information has finally surfaced as to their exact chemical nature and how damaging they can be. The amount of poison used is infinitesimal, but over time, like other food toxins, these minute doses build to quantities that can cause serious health problems.

Senator Ted Kennedy was among the first to try to prevent the cosmetic industry from being exempt from requiring warning labels on their toxic, commonly used products. The fact is that some of these substances are found in canned and packaged foods, as well as cosmetics.

If you knew one of the ingredients listed in your shampoo or deodorant is also contained in house paint and antifreeze - you would probably drop it like a smoldering coal. Most of us don't think about the fact that our skin is the largest organ of the body or that it quickly absorbs anything that's applied.

Most cosmetics contain Propylene Glycol which preserves anti-freeze, brake and hydraulic fluid, paints and coatings, floor wax and laundry detergent. It's also put into pet food, tobacco, baby wipes, toothpaste, shampoos, bubble bath, deodorants, lotions, processed foods and hundreds of other personal care items. It's found in every cream and cosmetic in the market place, even those you find in health food stores.

Propylene Glycol, prevents things from drying out. It keeps food items "delectably chewy" and keeps creams and lotions moist. It's been named by the American Academy of Dermatologist as a primary irritant causing a significant number of reactions. Even in low levels, it can cause contact dermatitis, kidney damage, liver abnormalities, rashes, dry skin and other skin abrasions. This is in addition to preventing and damaging cell growth and cell membranes, Propylene Glycol can be harmful by breathing the fumes, eating it or rubbing it into the skin. It's known to cause eye irritation, skin irritation, gastrointestinal problems, nausea, headache, vomiting and even depression.

A study from the U.S. Department of Health and Human Services National Toxicology Program pointed to DEA (diethanolamine) as being a carcinogenic preservative found in over 600 shampoos, conditioners, bubble baths, lotions, cosmetics, soaps, laundry and dish washing detergents. It has been proven to cause cancer when applied to the skin of rats.

Sodium Lauryl Sulfate, SLS is found in almost every shampoo and toothpaste on the market. Most commonly advertised cosmetic products have both SLS and Propylene Glycol.

SLS is used in concrete floor cleaners, engine de-greasers and car washing detergents. Classified as a mutagen, SLS is capable of changing genetic cell material. It actually corrodes hair follicles and impairs hair growth. When applied to the skin, it leaves residual material in the heart, liver, lungs, brain and can damage the immune system. It can also impede the natural development of children's eyes and cause permanent damage. (No wonder shampoo stings our eyes.)

There is often a warning label for children - especially for those under the age of two. These warnings are not to protect you or your children; they are designed to protect the manufacturers in the event of legal suits.

In the meantime, you might want to carry a magnifying glass in your purse or pocket to read the fine print on every label. Only purchase those with ingredients you recognize. Avoid cosmetics that contain: DEA, Propylene Glycol and Sodium Lauryl Sulfate. It's good to remember that canned and processed foods also include these ingredients, so it is vitally important to read the labels on everything. The accumulation of dyes, preservatives and food additives being absorbed at the same time, certainly contributes to the break down of cells and encourages cancer. Due to the growing awareness of these known carcinogens, there are now a growing number of chemical-free soaps, lotions and bath cosmetics. They are made from honey, coconut, olive oil and goat's milk and are much kinder to the body.

CHAPTER 18

VACCINES

~~~

INCREASING NUMBERS OF PEOPLE ARE learning about the dangers of vaccines and are refusing to vaccinate their children, which has stirred a great deal of controversy. Doctors warn that if children aren't vaccinated, we will see new outbreaks of measles, mumps, diphtheria, typhoid, polio, etc.

Years ago, childhood diseases like measles, mumps and chicken pox helped build the immune system, though not pleasant, they generally didn't kill anyone.

Diphtheria, typhoid and polio are more serious, but the way the vaccines are manufactured today, there are too many different disease strains given at the same time. An infant's developing immune system often can not tolerate this heavy bombardment and may suffer some serious deleterious effects.

There is huge body of evidence being denied by the allopathic medical profession indicating that vaccines are causing ADD, autism and other serious brain abnormalities. Despite their denial, these brain oriented problems are exploding exponentially and the emotional pain and financial burden that parents are having to endure is heartbreaking.

The National Institute of Health is still recommending vaccines, but the medical industry has been wrong many, many times. Due the the lack of long time testing, drugs are pulled from the market every year. With the rising instances of brain abnormalities like autism and ADD, pharmaceutical companies need to focus on finding safer ways to preserve vaccines that do not harm the brain and body as opposed to being indifferent to the heartbreak they continue to cause.

Although the whole mercury molecule was forced to be taken out of vaccines due to the known toxicity of mercury, vaccines are still preserved with a mercury derivative called thimerosol as well as formaldehyde, both of which are poisonous to the brain and body. This is in addition to many other harmful ingredients other than the disease itself. Is this what you want injecting into your new borns or toddlers who have not fully developed their immune systems?

Unless you are seeking the information from alternative researcher and newsletters, no one will tell you that many of the diseases we have today are manufactured in labs and distributed in vaccines to control population. If you don't believe it, you can research Ted which is an organization in San Francisco that invites geniuses to speak. In his 2014 lecture. Bill Gates, stated that he agreed with the method of controlling population through the use of vaccines.

In 1997, I interviewed a woman in Asheville, NC who had given birth to a beautiful, perfectly healthy boy. When she took him to the doctor for his check-up, he had a little cold. The doctor said he needed to get his DPT shot, but the mother said she would rather wait until his cold was gone. The doctor said, "Don't be ridiculous!" Despite her protest, he gave the baby the injection. The mother described her infant screaming all night like he was being stabbed. The next morning he was brain dead. Of course, the doctor was never held responsible.

Obviously, not everyone is going to have such a tragic reaction, but it makes one ponder whether it is worth taking the risk - especially when a child's immune system is threatened by a cold or fever.

In the 60's, I remember taking a typhoid shot in Chattanooga, when my husband and I were living there. They convinced us that there was a typhoid scare. Looking back today, that seems highly unlikely. After receiving my injection, I developed full blown typhoid, was deathly ill for over 6 weeks and have never taken a vaccine since. I always refuse flu shots and consistently observe those who do take them, still get the flu. Several nurses have shared with me privately, that they don't take flu shots either and neither do most doctors who are exposed daily to various forms of influenza.

CHAPTER 19

Electronic Pollution

I WOULD REMISS IF I didn't address the topic of ELF, Electric Low Frequency waves being radiated by all of the electronic tools in our lives. This includes: computers, Ipads, any kind of portable phones, cell phones, cell towers, kitchen appliances, microwave ovens, dimmer switches, televisions and the so-called "Smart Meters" that power companies utilize to monitor our use of electricity. These harmful frequencies are taking their toll on our bodies, particularly our nervous systems, yet the companies that manufacture, control and utilize them are in denial over their debatable "safe" use.

In the evolution of the human species, we are becoming more aware of the subtle unseen energies that exist in our lives. Until 50 or so years ago, you seldom heard the word vibration, today to hear someone say, "He has bad vibes or the house or restaurant has bad vibes is a common occurrence." We are so finely tuned that if an angry person comes into a room, without them saying a word, we immediately sense the anger frequencies emitting from their body.

Similar to trees, our bodies are highly sensitive electrical systems that react to changes in the electronic atmosphere. If trees are in proximity to high tension wires, they move their branches away or often die. When there is an upcoming cataclysm, whether it be a tornado, earthquake, volcanic eruption or a tsunami taking place thousands of miles away, before they occur, trees become very still as if holding their breath. If trees are sensitive enough to tune in to cataclysmic activity across the planet, it makes sense with the thousands of electrical networks that inundate our bodies, we have similar sensitivities. We all share the unified field of planet earth and within the last 50 years we are being bombarded by an accumulation of electronic frequencies that are foreign to our systems.

WHO, the World Health Organization, refuses to recognize that there are any proven health problems with electronic pollution, yet there are growing numbers of individuals who in the presence of ELF waves emitted from multiple sources are experiencing symptoms, the most common being chronic insomnia, pain or ringing in the ears, headaches, dizziness, memory loss, ADD, chronic fatigue, fibromyalgia, and other forms of face and brain pain. Electrical pollution aggravates preexisting conditions like MS and migraine headaches. Included in the research are the mounting statistics of brain cancer in adults and children.

Despite the arguments that the symptoms are often too mercurial to identify as being the cause, it's hard to deny when the sufferers move out of range of the electronic pollution, their symptoms cease.

Despite the statistics proving that people who live in proximity of high tension wires and cell towers are at a much higher risk of developing cancer, power companies continue to install more lines and towers to fit the needs of a public demanding better reception. Even with the increasing statistics of brain cancer, leukemia and other cancers among children, cell towers are now even installed on top of schools and churches. It's albeit impossible to escape the destructive frequencies they emit.

The University of California is among the institutions conducting research into the electronic pollution phenomenon. Their findings indicate ELF radiation could in fact be an international health threat, especially among children whose cell phone use is starting at an earlier and earlier age.

To be on the safe side of reasonable doubt, it's best to choose not to live close to high tension wires, cell towers or to keep cell phones anywhere on the body or even in the same room. The current large television entertainment rooms in American homes are definitely emitting radiation that few seem to recognize as harmful, as are the new cars that have sophisticated computer systems, GPS technology and TV's. This includes high technology offices where people are being bombarded with ELF waves from computers and other office machinery. In the meantime, thinking "ELF radiation won't affect me" is nothing less than naivete or denial. Whether you tend to believe you are being affected or not, pulling all of the plugs out at night before sleeping is an excellent way to reduce the harmful frequencies within the home.

I highly recommend, Dr. Robert Becker's two books on the subject, *Cross Currents* and *The Body Electric*. The National Foundation for Alternative Medicine is also an excellent source for providing current research into this growing new phenomenon threatening our health.

Part Two
Building the Immune System

*Drugs never cure a disease. They merely hush
the voice of nature's protest and pull down the
danger signals she erects. Any poison taken into
the system has to be reckoned with later. Pain
may disappear, but the patient is left in a worse
condition though unconscious of it at the time."*

Daniel Kress, MD

CHAPTER 20

THE IMPORTANCE OF DRINKING PURE WATER

DR. F. BATMANGHELIDJ'S IS A water researcher who began healing the body with just plain water. He contends, that because we don't drink just plain water, our bodies are literally suffering from draught and that many of the diseases we suffer can be healed with pure water. As a member of an organization calling for a new paradigm in healing called, *the Foundation for the Simple in Medicine,* his main contention is that our society is so product-oriented, that when we drink liquids, it's usually coffee, tea, juice or some kind of soda. We think these fluids are substitutes for water however, all of these drinks are highly acidic and open the door to inviting cancer cells.

It may sound overly simplistic, but when you read his reasoning backed by his research, it begins to make perfect sense. Dr. Batmanghelidj explains that we often do not pay attention to "the body's many cries for water" and most often, they are silenced with antacids or pain killers which he refers to as "pharmaceutical cocktails."

He explains that by the time the mouth is dry, the body is in an extreme state of dehydration and that noninfectious, recurring or chronic pain should first be viewed as indicators of body thirst. When blood becomes concentrated from lack of water, it draws water from the surrounding cells causing dehydration in various parts of the body, often causing pain.

Published in the *Journal of Clinical Gastroenterology*, June 1983, the doctors's report explains his water therapy success with over 3,000 people. He describes his positive results with dyspeptic pain, colitis, rheumatism, arthritis, anginal pain, low back pain, leg pain, migraines, chronic fatigue, hangovers and many others.

He says, "My book, *Your Bodies Many Cries for Water,* is a preventive and self-education manual for those who prefer to adhere to the logic of the natural and the simple in medicine."

Because of our dependence on sweet tastes, Dr. B explains that when the body becomes dehydrated, humans seem to lose their thirst sensation, often not recognizing their need for water and will gravitate toward something sweet. He describes the many roles that water plays in the body, including lubricating joints, digestion, feeding the spinal fluids and providing adhesive in cell architecture.

In addition, to flushing out the liver and kidneys, water contributes greatly to beautiful skin by preventing acne and other skin out breaks. It's most important job is igniting the electrical charge that carries energies to the cells.

Dr. B cites many of his healing successes with just water, but one in particular stands out. A young man had been suffering from ulcers. When the doctor was called in, he was doubled over in pain and semiconscious on the floor. Shaking him to get a response, the doctor learned he had already taken three tables of cimetidine and a whole bottle of antacid without any relief. The doctor feared the patient might have "acute abdomen" or a perforated ulcer requiring surgical exploration. Feeling the abdominal wall for rigidity, he determined that this wasn't the case and decided to treat the patient with water.

When he suggested the patient drink two glasses of water, he responded with great hesitation. The doctor then said to him, "You have taken the usual medications without any result. Now, why don't you try my suggestion?"

The man drank the two glasses of water. In fifteen minutes his pain had become less severe and his groaning stopped. The doctor gave him another glass of water and in a few moments, the pain disappeared completely. It had taken three glasses of water and a total of 20 minutes. **Dr. B suggests that gastritis, duodenitis and heartburn should be treated with water alone.** In the case of an ulcer - the addition of a change of diet.

Your Body's Many Cries for Water offers a wonderful explanation of how vital water is to our health and the many physical ills that have benefited from the following simple suggestions.

* Drink an absolute minimum of six to eight 8 oz. glasses of water a day.

(Alcohol, coffee, tea, and caffeine-containing beverages absolutely **do not** count as water.)

* The best regimen to follow is to drink one 8 oz. glass, one half-hour before taking meals and a similar amount two and one half hours after each meal. Two glasses should be taken before your heaviest meal and before going to bed.

CHAPTER 21

Proper Breathing

OF ALL FUNCTIONS OF OUR body, our breath is the most important. The lungs are the main engine of the body and our breath is the most important of any bodily function. We can go without food for 30 days, without water for 3 days, but we die after three minutes without breath. Our breath carries oxygen to the cells and brain, controls our physical and mental equilibrium and balances both the sympathetic and parasympathetic systems. It has been proven that cancer cannot exist in a highly oxygenated environment.

Taking the time to be aware of the rhythm of our breathing and trying to take slow deliberate breaths deep into our stomach, such as is taught by authentic Yoga systems, can result in major improvements in our health. Stress can be controlled on a daily basis by being aware of when we hold our breath, forget to breathe, or breathe in an accelerated fashion.

My son, Ross Kamens is a restaurant consultant, nutritional expert and Yoga instructor. Last year when he was visiting, we were rushing around running errands. He stopped and said, "Mom, you are not breathing. Slow down and breathe."

With all of the Yoga and workshops I've done over the years, I knew the importance of breathing. But, there I was, so caught up in the self-imposed stress of the moment, I was unconscious of the fact that I was holding my breath. My response was, "You're right son. Thanks for reminding me."

Deliberate, steady breathing is a profound method that can create giant leaps in emotional, physical and spiritual wellness. It's important to note some of the pioneers in the breath movement.

In 1990, Judith Kravitz emerged calling her method, *Transformational Breathing*. She later founded, The International Breath Institute, to study breath and educate the public as to the many applications for creating physical and mental health. Proper breathing can lower stress, lower blood pressure, calm the nervous system and place the body in a more balanced state conducive to overall well being and the restoration of poor health. Years ago, that was the original function of spas, they were situated in nature, amidst non-polluted mountain springs or ocean resorts where one could breathe properly and drink pure water.

As is taught in all forms of traditional Yoga, breathing literally is the staff of life and if practiced deliberately, it can provide enhanced thinking, physical performance and a can facilitate a pathway to spiritual awakening.

In the field of Transpersonal Psychology, Stanislov Grof, a Harvard Ph.D. discovered he could stimulate visions and revelations with the use of accelerated breathing. He and his wife Christine, began a trademark system called, *Holotropic Breath Work*. Typical of the breathing methods utilized by ancient Shamans to elevate energy and consciousness, Dr. Grof is able to guide people into the higher revelatory states that were once practiced by ancient societies more advanced than our own.

Thanks to a deeper knowledge of the importance of regulated breathing, childbirth can be a more healthy, loving experience. With the wonderful influence of the *La Maze* method and the practices of mid-wives, by utilizing a specific system of breathing, babies are delivered naturally, then gently eased on to their mother's stomach. There is no toxic anesthesia used, nor is there a harsh disconnect from the mother who begins immediately nurturing and nursing her child. Physically and spiritually, this is an infinitely more tender, caring and enlightened way to bring children into the world than using any kind of drug or unnecessary surgery.

Unfortunately today, Caesarian births are occurring with increasing frequency, and more often than not, are scheduled for the convenience of the obstetrician, as opposed to when the baby itself is ready to be born naturally.

CHAPTER 22

FRESH, LOCALLY GROWN FOODS CONTAIN VITAL ENZYMES

THE BEST REASON FOR EATING organic foods is that they taste better and are loaded with the enzymes needed for digestion. You can readily see the difference in the freshly grown foods sold at the locally grown organic farmer's markets that are cropping up all over the country. Not only do the foods give off a ripe, colorful, radiant energy, they have actual old-fashioned flavor like many of us remember when we were children.

If fruits and vegetable do not have a healthy color, it's a good indication that they simply are not balanced nutritionally, are old or have been heavily sprayed. It's best to avoid them. Too many of the fruits and vegetables in markets are shipped from long distances from foreign countries. They're picked green, often tasteless and low in food value. I'm sure you have tried tomatoes in super markets that have a pale, anemic color and taste like predigested styrofoam.

Regardless of TV chefs who come up with easy-to-prepare recipes, or the sales propaganda persuading you about the convenience of packaged or frozen foods, they simply do not have the food value of freshly grown fruits and vegetables. In the canning process, chemicals like MSG and BHT, Nagalese and Propylene Glycol are added to preserve the foods. The canning process itself destroys the live enzymes and nutrients vital to the healthy functioning of your organs and immune system.

As opposed to being sprayed with toxic pesticides and herbicides, organic soil has a higher mineral and enzyme count because the soil is nurtured with organic materials including: composted fruits and vegetables; iron-filled garden weeds; crop residue; cow manure and other natural minerals and enzymes. Rudolph Steiner, the father of Bio-Dynamic gardening discovered that cow manure has a special enzyme necessary for human digestion but today, cow manure is rarely used on corporate farms.

Enzymes are essential to life and fresh organically grown vegetables and fruits simply contain more live enzymes. These nutrients do not exist in foods grown in depleted soil sprayed with pesticides and herbicides or in those foods undergoing the freezing necessary to transport them.

Humans have a limited amount of digestive enzymes - protease to digest protein, amylase to digest starch and lipase that digests fats. If we continue to eat cooked, processed foods, or fruits that are not fully ripe, our ability to digest becomes dramatically hampered, particularly as we get older. Live enzymes play a significant role in any healing process. When experiencing gas, bloating, heart burn or any kind of indigestion, rather than relying on over-the-counter digestive aids, taking digestive enzymes is a healthier way to handle most digestive problems. Enzymes are so important, many holistic physicians utilize enzyme therapy in the healing of cancer.

Pioneer physicians like Dr. Gabriel Cousins, author of *Conscious Eating* and Chemist-Nutritionist Dr. Lita Lee of *Grassroots Network* agree that minerals are the essential catalysts that trigger the function of vitamins and enzymes. If we do not have minerals in the soil as a catalyst for enzymes, they can't do their job of carrying life producing energy to the blood stream. Many families and communities in America are now planting their own organic gardens to make sure they're getting all of these important nutrients and enzymes necessary to improving their family's health.

Raw foods have the most live enzymes and it's important to have a raw salad with your meals. But, if you do decide to try all raw foods, it's wise to proceed slowly, it can cause digestive complications. With any meal, if you observe how you feel after you've eaten, (especially the next day), and you find you are feeling sluggish or tired, you can usually attribute your condition to what you ate the night before. If you consistently observe how your body feels after every meal and avoid those things that produce gas, bloating or fatigue, your body will actually begin craving the foods you need.

There are many greens that have different tastes such as chard, bok choy, spinach, cabbage, even brussels sprouts that if chopped can provide delicious salad combinations. For vegetarians, adding raw walnuts, almonds and cashews helps to provide protein. Sesame, poppy, pumpkin and other seeds provide protein as well.

For most people, it's best to eat raw in the summer and more cooked foods in winter. Summer crops produce cooling foods like fruits, berries, avocados, mushrooms and melons. In the winter, we need root vegetables and hot soups that provide heat in our bodies. Combining hearty, warming soups with a raw salad is a good way to have a balanced meal.

If you have a hard time finding ways to include winter greens in your diet, one of the simplest and quickest ways to prepare, collards, chard, spinach, kale and other greens is to steam them. When they're done, sprinkle them with olive oil, lemon juice and a little vegetable or sea salt. They are delicious and seldom taste slimy or overcooked.

An easy way to have nutritional balance is to choose foods of varying colors. Each color has a different nutrient that your body needs at those specific times of the year. To get the idea, picture a salad with yellow peppers, purple cabbage, red tomatoes along with your favorite salad greens. You will have a colorful combination that's also very healthy.

According to Dr. Bernard Jensen, one of original leaders in the holistic movement, "The best way to feed your body live fresh enzymes is by drinking freshly squeezed juices."

Freshly squeezed is important because the longer the juice is exposed to air, the less enzymes it has. Don't let anyone tell you that bottled juices still have the same level of enzymes, they don't. If you drink juices regularly, you soon learn to taste the difference. Carrot juice is one of the most highly recommended because of its high content of beta-carotene that fights cancer. If you are not a carrot juice lover, you can add apple, celery, cucumber or a number of other interesting combinations to make it more palatable.

When juicing, some kind of blue/green algae or a chlorophyl product can add to the process of getting the green nutrients that build the body and purify the blood stream. If you have a hard time eating greens, which many people do, putting actual raw greens into your smoothy is a wonderful way to camouflage the taste. Many raw food nutritionists promote wheat grass juice that has a high concentration of chlorophyll and is very healing for the body.

Health oriented juice bars are now a permanent fixture in most communities. They offer a number of delicious combinations. Along with fresh, ripe, organically grown foods and raw salads, juicing really is one of the fastest and easiest ways to build up the body's own storehouse of enzymes.

CHAPTER 23

THE CHALLENGE OF PROPER FOOD COMBINING

YEARS AGO, HARVEY AND MARILYN Diamond's book, *Fit for Life* came on to the market. They were the first to discuss the idea of proper food combining. Selling over twelve million copies worldwide, *Fit for Life* not only introduced a new dining paradigm, it impacted more people than any other diet book. The Diamonds closely followed the research of Nobel prize winning Russian scientist Ivan Pavlov and natural hygienist Dr. Herbert Shelton who many years ago, espoused the theory of proper food combining as a way to induce perfect health. At the time of their discoveries, the medical world was not ready to consider the idea that disease could be caused by eating improperly, however, the evidence is now insurmountable. With the abundance of statistics pointing directly to our food source as the cause of many major diseases, the media is consumed with addressing the kind and quality of foods we consume. However, because the information is often just hyping diet courses or delicious sounding recipes, we need to be aware of what really adheres to proper food combining.

With exception of a handful of natural foods doctors and healers like Drs. Max Gerson and Herbert Shelton, there was never a true science of food. We tended to eat what was available with little discretion. Since Americans presently spend over $2 billion a year on antacids and digestive aids, you might want to take a more serious look at food combining.

One of the reasons the *"Fit for Life"* diet became popular was because dieters could eat large quantities of food and still lose weight. Most of us are not as active as our ancestors who did laborious farming and building. We live much more sedentary lives and simply do not need as many of the carbohydrates. If people integrate the rules into their daily diet, they will experience the bonus of weight loss and their indigestion problems disappear. Poor food combining prevents food nutrients from being properly absorbed into the system.

The basic theory is simple. Certain foods require specific acid or alkaline digestive juices to be properly absorbed by the stomach. All proteins, meat, fish, dairy and nuts require an acid digestive juice.

Starches such as bread, pasta, grains, potatoes and cereal require an alkaline digestive juice. We don't have to be chemists to know that acid and alkaline neutralize each other. If we eat foods from both categories, our food spoils in the stomach causing various types of indigestive discomfort, bloating, lethargy, fat and in extreme cases malnutrition.

No matter how small the portions of food we eat during Thanksgiving and Christmas, we walk away from the table bloated and uncomfortable. If you consume meats, starch, fruit, sugar, vegetables and alcohol at the same time as cream, butter, oils, gravies, fats, nuts, cheese and eggs, according to Dr. Shelton, you've created the gastronomical torture chamber that most of us have experienced.

The General rules of proper food combining are:

Eat proteins with vegetables.
Eat grains with vegetables.
Eat fruit alone.
Dairy, fats and oils should not be consumed with meat.
Sugar should NEVER be eaten with protein.
Milk should be taken alone or not at all.

As you can see, even though they might taste great, most of the American diet is terrible food combining.

Our often favorite combinations are; meat and potatoes, fish and rice; chicken with noodles or rice; eggs and toast; milk and nuts; beans or bread with cheese; cereal and milk. Any kind of sandwich is poor food combining and the cause of a great deal of stress to the system.

Two proteins should not be consumed at the same time such as: bacon and eggs or cheeseburgers. Single protein meals assure greater digestive efficiency. Due to the high alkaline factor of fruit, and the digestion time it requires, it should **always** be eaten alone and at least 30 minutes before or three hours after a meal. Mixing fruit with the other ingredients that go into a holiday meal is like adding a match to the bomb.

It's also good to know that some fruits don't even combine well with each other. Melon, citrus and bananas are always best eaten alone or they will putrefy in the stomach causing gas and bloating.

Most food combining advocates agree that cooked apple is an exception. Because of having an almost neutral PH, it can be eaten with either starch or proteins. However, apple combined with corn will sometimes cause difficulty. Another exception is banana. Because of its starchy consistency, bananas combine well with other starches which makes banana bread a fairly good option for dessert.

The other strict rule is the "No, No" about milk. Milk combines poorly with all other foods because it coagulates forming curds that surround other food particles insulating them against the gastric juices. This delays the digestion of other foods until after the milk curds dissipate.

For many of us, the most difficult rule of food combining is to eat starch and sugar at separate meals. Sugar is known to not only leech B vitamins from the body, it hinders the digestion of protein. Sugar and beans in the same meal is like a nuclear bomb in your stomach. The same is true for eating dessert at the end of a meal. According to Dr. Shelton, "if you must eat a piece of pie, eat the pie and a large raw vegetable salad and nothing else - and then miss the next meal."

If you eat fruit with something - nuts and seeds are the most compatible. But remember the citrus, melon and banana exceptions. Unsalted raw almonds, hulled sunflower, sesame seeds and pumpkin seeds ground and sprinkled over fruit work best.

Good protein combinations include: fish and vegetables, baked chicken and steamed vegetables or egg and vegetable omelets.

Celebrity chefs are famous for adding fruits as a decoration to meat dishes. It's better to garnish with raw vegetables rather than fruits. As stated before, fruits and vegetables should NEVER be eaten together. So all of those sexy raw salads with pears, berries and raisins present a challenge to your digestive system. Most vegetables combine well with proteins, but because of its high fat content, avocado is the exception. It does not combine well with meat or nuts.

For meat and potato eaters who think food combining is bunk, it's been noted by natural hygienists that animals in nature eat only one food type at a time.

CHAPTER 24

Support For the Immune System

We often don't realize that the skin is the largest organ of the body and is one of the natural dumping grounds for the liver. If you have acne, a rash or an outbreak of any kind, it's a signal that your liver is toxic and needs cleaning.

Dry brushing your skin with a good strong brush seems like such an insignificant thing to do, but before getting into the shower, it's a great way to stimulate the blood stream. It helps carry toxins from the liver out of the pores.

When showering, the Native Americans have a simple thing they do daily that helps build the immune system. At the end of your warm shower, turn on the cold water for a few minutes. It's not easy to do at first, but you'll find that it immediately provides a natural jolt of energy. It stimulates the thyroid and immune system strengthening your body for the onslaught of toxins that we confront daily. Remember most rivers and streams have a cold temperature, so there's good reason for drinking or bathing in cold water.

Drinking the juice of a lemon in hot water every morning is a way to detox your liver and put your body in an alkaline state. Deepak Chopra suggests strait lemon juice in the morning building up to 12 lemons and then going back down to one lemon a day to completely detoxify your liver.

Doing a few exercises first thing in the morning to stimulate all of your organs is important. Even 10 to 20 minutes of easy stretching helps. Yoga, is an excellent way to bring oxygen to the cells and organs. There are many easy postures and breathing exercises that almost anyone can do. The Yoga posture called, the *Salute to the Sun*, is often referred to as the perfect morning exercise.

Fasting is an excellent way to detox the body and give your overall system a rest. Many stomach problems can be helped by fasting. There's a number of excellent juice fasts that you can do at home and formulas that can be obtained at your local health food store. There's usually someone on the staff that can guide you to the formula that's best for you. If you are interested, it's a good idea to do some research before you start so you don't detox too quickly. A combination of fasting and colon cleansing is highly beneficial to your health

CHAPTER 25

The Healing Power of Vitamin C

You know how vitamins sit on our shelf and we forget to take them, Vitamin C is one of those often taken for granted, but it is one with a long, outstanding, proven history of success. I attribute much of my good health to my daily use of Vitamin C and the fact that when I'm feeling an oncoming cold or flu, I increase my dosage to five or six thousand milligrams a day.

In 1937, after seeing a scientific report, Merck Laboratories ran an ad in the *AMA Journal*, December 17, 1938 encouraging the use of Vitamin C exclaiming the anti-viral and anti-toxic properties. However, shortly afterwards, sulfa and penicillin came in to use and Vitamin C was disregarded in favor of the more expensive "wonder drugs."

With exception of doctors suggesting to "drink orange juice," Vitamin C didn't become popular again until 1973 when Dr. Linus Pauling released his book, *Vitamin C and the Common Cold*. Pauling suggested 4 to 10 grams daily starting at the first symptom continuing each day as necessary. Depending on weight, size and other factors, 10 to 15 grams a day were suggested as safe.

Dentist Stephen Sheffrey, of Ann Arbor, Michigan released a booklet to educate the public about the value of C. If administered in large enough doses, he cited successes in cases of allergies, asthma, chronic fatigue, shingles, hepatitis, tumors, colon polyps, clogged arteries and even cancer and strokes.

Dr. Sheffrey explains, "20% of the population is allergic to Vitamin C. They experience side effects such as sore mouth, rash, excess gas, cramps and diarrhea. Conversely, eighty percent of the population can take 10 to 15 grams in divided doses and even more when ill. Among the 80% group, diarrhea only occurs when C isn't needed, when too much is taken per dose, or when taken on an empty stomach." Sheffrey explains that the research into Vitamin C for serious diseases failed, either because doses were not high enough or not administered intravenously.

In 1971, Cancer Specialist, Dr. Ewan Cameron of Boston, Mass. began giving his cancer patients Vitamin C injections and became convinced that for certain patients, Vitamin C is better than the toxic effects of chemotherapy or radiation that tends to breakdown the whole immune system. Many holistic physicians hoped his evidence would have prompted scientific research on the use of intravenous C for lymphatic and other types of cancer. Unfortunately it hasn't. Since Vitamin C is such an inexpensive drug to use, it doesn't inspire research for use by large pharmaceutical companies. They are not in a hurry to find an inexpensive or pain-free way to heal cancer. Instead, they favor a number of procedures and medications accompanying chemo and radiation treatments that help escalate those huge hospital bills.

CHAPTER 26

COLLOIDAL SILVER AND ITS ANTIBIOTIC PROPERTIES

WITH THE INTRODUCTION OF ANTIBIOTICS and environmental estrogens into our livestock, farm animals now receive dosages of antibiotics thirty times higher than humans. These additives remain in our meat and milk which now contain some 80 different chemicals. As a result of high levels of food ingested antibiotics, a study at Rutgers University reported that resistant bacteria has increased from 600 to 2700 per cent rendering most antibiotics ineffective against resistant bacteria and various diseases. MRSA and Morgellons are examples of these resistant strains that are increasing daily in hospitals. Pharmaceutical drugs are responsible for causing a number of new diseases referred to as Iatrogenics.

Because of the overuse of antibiotics, holistic practitioners are now returning to various herbs and ancient remedies that have been proven to work over the centuries. One of the most effective among these is colloidal silver.

Silver has been used medicinally for over 1200 years. The famous German physician Paracelsus was one of the first to understand the broad spectrum healing qualities of colloidal silver. He relied on silver as a highly effective antiseptic and antibiotic using it to cure all kinds of viral, skin and nerve diseases.

Most of us are familiar with the silver goblet traditionally used during the communion sacrament. Long recognized by nobility for killing bacteria, one contact with silver and liquids will retain their antiseptic quality even after contact no longer exists. In India, China and countries around the world, there are hundreds of examples of the use of silver to retard spoilage in milk and other foods. Today, sheets of silver are often served in India as a gourmet delicacy.

Colloidal silver was rediscovered in the 1800's and prior to 1938 was administered in just about every way that modern drugs are used. In addition to being dropped into the eyes; it was injected both intravenously and intramuscularly. It was used as a gargle for throat conditions, taken orally, and applied topically for sensitive tissues and was even used as a douche.

In was in the 1940's when it was disregarded in favor of the new "cure all" antibiotics which, at that time were less expensive. Unlike antibiotics, which encourage drug resistant strains, silver kills harmful pathogens on contact. Few known virus, bacteria, fungus or parasites can exist within the presence of even minute traces of silver. Occurring naturally in the body, it's known to combat at least 650 harmful bacterial strains. To date, there is no evidence of germs developing resistance or immunity to silver.

Richard L. Davies, is the Executive Director of the Silver Institute in Washington, DC. He monitors silver technology in 37 countries. "In four years, we discovered 87 important new medical uses for silver," says Davies. We're just beginning to see what extent it can relieve suffering and save lives."

In 1919, Alfred Searle of Searle Laboratories wrote, "The germicidal action of certain metals in the colloidal state has been demonstrated in a large number of human cases with astonishingly successful results. For internal administration, either orally or hypodermically, they have the advantage of being rapidly fatal to the parasites both bacterial and otherwise, without any toxic action on the host."

Despite these profound results, silver has never been encouraged in favor of more profit generating antibiotics.

In his research, Dr. Robert Becker, author of *The Body Electric* discovered a correlation between chronically ill people and the absence of low levels of silver in their blood. He concluded that their absence accounted for a lowered immune system and that it stimulated the growth of injured tissue, eliminated diseased cells and discouraged the presence of cancer cells.

Colloidal silver is an antiseptic, antibacterial and antiviral substance that heals bronchial infections, eye infections and most of the new viruses. For those suffering from Candida or antibiotic allergies, it's an excellent alternative. Good quality colloidal silver can be purchased in health food stores. The darker solutions are much more effective than those created by home made colloidal silver making machines.

Olive leaf is also known for it's antiviral and antibiotic properties. Used in combination with Colloidal Silver, they are known to eradicate serious diseases such as bronchitis and other deep viral or bacterial infections. There are no side affects and are much safer to use than the current antibiotics relied upon by most allopathic physicians.

CHAPTER 27

COLON CLEANSING

MOST OF US ARE NOT aware that if you have a truly healthy colon, you should be having a bowel movement after every meal. However, with the consumption of junk foods, sugar, wheat, canned and frozen foods, that isn't the case for most people. They are happy if they have one bowel movement a day, and some people only have one a week.

Colon cleansing is a repulsive topic for many people, but if you are a meat eater, it is particularly important because meat digests slowly in the gut. If your bowels aren't regular, toxins from the rotting meat and undigested foods collect on the sides of your colon often producing parasites. A good indicator of toxins or parasites is a bulging stomach.

Similar to enemas, colon cleansing is a method of using water and derma-massage to flush out any old fecal debris. It's painless and in many cases will not only eliminate a bloated stomach, it will help to remove parasites and eliminate clouded thinking. You will be shocked to see what comes out of your body and how much has been stored.

According to two of America's famous herbalists Hannah Kroger and Hulda Clark, "parasites are the precursor to cancer." It's important to go in for colonics regularly and is one of the best things you can do to prevent cancer.

It is also important to take herbs to kill parasites. Just like dogs and cats, humans also have worms, and it's important to occasionally take an herbal formula to remove them. A combination of wormwood, clove and black walnut is a popular formula. Among holistic practitioners. taking three of each, three times a day is a helpful regimen.

I'd been living in one of the most remote areas of Mexico for about five months. Several months after returning home, I was having trouble sleeping and one of my friends suggested I take wormwood five days before the full moon and then 4 days afterward to help me sleep. I nearly fainted when I passed a two foot long black worm that looked like a snake.

Years later, I used a micro-current machine and set it on the parasite protocol. The very next morning, I passed hundreds of tiny white worms about an inch long. Again I was shocked. A few weeks later, I did it again and passed the mother and father of those little white devils and they were over two feet long. I couldn't believe it.

Colon therapy is not encouraged by allopathic physicians, but it's an excellent way to rid your body of toxins by stimulating the liver. In holistic clinics, coffee enemas are used daily to stimulate the cleansing of the liver, particularly for cancer victims. There are good colon therapists in every city. Asking around at health food stores is a good way to locate the best ones.

CHAPTER 28

MEDICINAL SPICES USED IN COOKING

IN ADDITION TO BEING A natural way of eliminating parasites, culinary herbs came into use by earlier cultures for both their healing benefits and to enhance flavor. Most of us, at one time or another have used oregano and cinnamon, but haven't considered that they might have healing, antiseptic attributes. These particular culinary herbs are extremely helpful in keeping the immune system stimulated.

Garlic is one of the body's great blood purifiers and has antibiotic properties. It provides a great defense against colds and flu and also kills parasites that invade the colon. The more garlic you eat, the better off you are.

Internationally recognized physician Dr. Dietrich Klinghardt encourages the use of culinary herbs. He says, "Don't be afraid to use larger amounts of the herbs suggested in recipes. If they're not freshly grown, they've lost most of their potency. Even if they're fresh, the more you use, the better it is for the immune system." Most culinary herbs today are now radiated which lowers their life force and effectiveness. It's best to grow your own.

According to Dr. Klinghardt, both oregano and cilantro are excellent anti-bacterials. Oregano leaves are one of the most common herbs used in America however, the oil is now commonly suggested by many alternative practitioners to rid bacterial infections. Oregano is used in all Italian and Greek recipes and, is perhaps one of the reasons why the Mediterranean diet has been favored as being the most healthful.

For some, cilantro is a taste that has to be developed, but it is a diverse herb traditionally used in both Mexican, East Indian and Thai food. Becoming more widely used by American chefs and gourmet cooks, it's being added to baked meats and salads. If you haven't tried cilantro before, there are recipes that can be found on the Internet that include this highly, antibacterial herb.

With the increase in the East Indian population in America, we're becoming more familiar with Indian culinary herbs. Turmeric has been proven to deter cancer. Turmeric contains curcumin, a therapeutic ingredient that has antioxidant, anti-inflammatory, antiseptic and analgesic properties that boost the immune system. It also helps control cholesterol levels, is a liver detoxifier that regulates metabolism and weight management. This is in addition to improving memory and brain function. Turmeric also helps skin conditions, neurological disorders and lowers triglycerides. By adding black pepper to turmeric or turmeric-spiced food, the body's absorption rate is increased by 2000%. If you wish to take turmeric as a cancer preventive, it can be obtained in capsules at health food stores.

Used since ancient Egypt, Cinnamon is now recognized for being an anti-viral herb. According to the U.S. National Library of Medicine, Cinnamon is used to help treat colds, sore throats, arthritis, muscle spasms, vomiting, diarrhea, infections, loss of appetite, and erectile dysfunction. It also lowers the negative effects of meals high in fat.

According to England's *Diabetes UK* magazine, cinnamon may lower blood sugar and lipids in people with type 1 or type 2 diabetes. *The National Institute of Health* reports that cinnamaldehyde, a chemical found in Cassia cinnamon can help fight against bacterial and fungal infections. Professor Michael Ovadia of the Department of Zoology at Tel Aviv University discovered that an extract found in cinnamon bark contains properties that can inhibit the development of Alzheimer's.

Honey is another one of nature's medicinal substances that can bring healing to many parts of the body. Dr. Robert Hawk, was a gynecological surgeon at Transylvania Hospital in Brevard, NC. While serving as a Chief Resident of Obstetrics and Gynecology at Charlotte Memorial Hospital. He was assigned a patient who after cancer surgery had developed gangrene that was so serious, the foul smell of decaying flesh had permeated her room and he was in a quandary as to what to do to help her. That week, he happened to pick up a copy of an Australian medical journal with an article discussing the healing power of honey. Dr. Hawk was so impressed by the information, he decided he had nothing to lose and gave the nurses instructions to apply honey to the woman's wounds three times a day.

"The nurses thought I'd had lost my mind and all of my colleagues in the hospital thought I'd turned loony. Think about it, honey is a food product that never spoils," said Dr. Hawk. "It never decomposes. There is obviously something in it that deters bacteria."

His courage and intuition proved to be correct. The day after applying the honey to the infected incisions, the odor was gone from the room and the patient was released 7 days later. After that experience, he applied honey to the incisions of all of his surgery patients and the nurse who worked with him attested to the fact that he was the only doctor at Transylvania hospital who never had a patient develop any post-op infections. He was finally exonerated several later when Johns Hopkins conducted a lecture series about honey being an excellent healer for wounds and incisions.

Dr. Hawk's story allowed me to be open to the follow information about the healing powers of both honey and cinnamon which are in their own category. Their healing powers seem endless.

* It's commonly suggested that those suffering from common or severe colds should take one tablespoon honey with 1/4 tablespoon cinnamon powder daily for three days. This process will deliciously cure most chronic cough, colds and clear the sinuses. For a throat tickle or

raspy voice, take one tablespoon of honey and sip until gone. Repeat every three hours until the throat is without symptoms.

The glucose content of honey is infinitely more heathy for the body than sugar. When taken in the right dosage as a medicine, it is not harmful to diabetic patients. By simply eating honey and cinnamon on toast, instead of fruit preserves, the combination reduces cholesterol along with strengthening and revitalizing arteries and veins preventing heart attacks.

Copenhagen University found that when doctors treated their patients with a mixture of one tablespoon honey and half teaspoon cinnamon powder before breakfast, within a week, 73 out of the 200 arthritic patients were totally relieved of pain. Within a month, almost all the patients who were not ambulatory, started walking without pain.

Learning about these simple, inexpensive culinary herbs readily found and inexpensively purchased can add so many health benefits to our lives. Something as simple as increasing our use of honey, instead of sugar, and recognizing the medicinal properties of these ancient culinary herbs is a good start. It makes sense to integrate them into our diet.

Epilogue

After 30 years of research and observation, I truly believe that nature has provided everything we need to heal ourselves. It's sad that our current medical profession has ignored many of the simple and natural healing methods that our ancestors practiced. The pharmaceutical industry that funds and controls most of the medical schools have purposely kept this information out of the marketplace in favor of costly medications and procedures. They do not practice preventive medicine and no longer teach the natural, pain-free things that will not reap large profits.

The accumulation of GMO's, food and water additives, preservatives, pesticides, food dyes, toxic metals and various air and frequency pollutants contribute greatly to the rise of cancer and the other so-called incurable diseases now plaguing our society. Keeping the body free of these harmful things is vital. We simply can not rely on our government to safeguard us, we must take a proactive role in protecting ourselves. It's important to understand that those who control our health, control our lives.

The things I've listed as being those to avoid or to add to your daily routines may seem overwhelming. They obviously can't be included all at once. You can begin by thinking about the things that are the easiest for you to do, and then start with what you feel you can handle. It's a learning process. It's worth making the extra effort to avoid having your breasts cut off, prostate surgery, organs removed, brain tumors or having any kind of debilitating chemo or radiation. I've painfully observed the horrible suffering that accompanies these options among my family and friends. I consistently avoid most of the commonly accepted prescription medicines and procedures by choosing natural remedies. If we stay as close to nature as we possibly can, our chances of increasing our good health and longevity are greatly enhanced and the possibilities of getting cancer are dramatically reduced. Your being willing to try to change how you view the foods you are eating and the choices you make can save your own life, and the lives of your family.

> ***"Let Your Food Be Your Medicine and***
> ***Your Medicine Be Your Food."***
>
> **HIPPOCRATES**

Made in the USA
San Bernardino, CA
24 August 2017